The Diverticulitis

Handbook

How to Live Pain Free

Foods to Eat & Avoid
3 Phase Diet Guide
21 Recipe Cookbook
Index of Causes and Symptoms

by

ELIZABETH GRAY

Copyright © 2017 by Elizabeth Gray

ISBN-13:
978-1979648127
ISBN-10:
1979648123

Elizabeth Gray Publishing
18 Key Street
Millis, MA 02054

"Let food be thy medicine and medicine be thy food."

~ HIPPOCRATES

DISCLAIMER

The information in this book does not contain medical professional advice. Individuals requiring such services should consult a competent medical professional. The author makes no representations about the suitability of the information contained in this book for any purpose. This material is provided "as is" and this publication is for informational purposes only.

TABLE OF CONTENTS

INTRODUCTION

Why am I writing this book? It's simple really. To help others self-educate with this increasingly common disease. Diverticulitis is becoming more common and I have known family members and friends who have been diagnosed with the disease. It is especially important to have a background of diverticulitis when you're a caregiver for someone with a health issue.

Diverticulitis is very painful and no fun to live with. People may not know they have it at all until they go to the emergency room or to their primary doctor. Most know there's something wrong. As the saying goes "trust your gut". This holds true more than ever to people diagnosed with diverticulitis.

This handbook covers the disease basics, history, symptoms, treatment, foods to avoid, lifestyle changes, and the diverticulitis diet with simple recipes. I strongly encourage you to see your physician if you believe you have any signs of the disease. With this handbook and the help of your physician, living with diverticulitis will become easier. You will be less anxious and less stressed for a reason: you will have all of the dietary and other specialized knowledge you need to eventually tame those diverticulitis uncomfortable spells once and for all.

What Is Diverticulitis
vs. Diverticulosis?

To get started we need to go over the various terms used to describe diverticulitis.

- Diverticular Disease
  This is an umbrella term for both diverticulosis and diverticulitis. Basically, *diverticulosis* does not have any symptoms and people may not know they even have it until they have a *diverticulosis* flare up. Diverticular disease includes a spectrum of conditions ranging from asymptomatic diverticular disease (with no symptoms), to symptomatic uncomplicated diverticular disease (with few problems), and complicated diverticular disease that includes acute and chronic *diverticulitis* (with flare ups)

- Diverticulosis
  Basically diverticulosis means having *diverticula* in your system, small pouches or sacs that form in the wall of the large intestine or colon. These bulge outward through weak spots.

- Diverticulitis
  If these *diverticula* become inflamed or infected a *diverticulitis* flare up exists. While the colon is the most common area to get *diverticulitis*, the *diverticula*

can form anywhere for example in the throat, esophagus, stomach, and small intestine.

While not true in every case, age plays a big role in diverticulosis. Over 40 years of age, diverticula are common in an estimated 10 percent of the U.S. population. Approximately half of Americans over the age of 60 have diverticula somewhere in their digestive organs. By age 80, an estimated 65 percent of people have diverticulitis. Often older people too are taking drugs which suppress the immune system which also increases the risk of colon infection and diverticulitis.

While these diverticula (pouches) usually don't cause problems, for those whose diverticula do, people will experience inflammation and even a massive painful infection. The symptoms are similar to those of appendicitis, except the pain is usually in the lower-left side of your abdomen rather than the lower right. Less common signs include nausea, vomiting, unexplained fever and chills, bloating and gas, rectal bleeding, frequent or difficulty with urination, persistent diarrhea or constipation, recurring urinary tract infections. If you start having any symptom of diverticulitis, call your doctor right away. Untreated diverticulitis can lead to dangerous complications.

Summary

Diverticulosis is when you have the presence of diverticula. If the diverticula becomes infected, you have diverticulitis. Once you quell the diverticulitis outbreak, you return to having benign or asymptomatic diverticulitis. If you can maintain diverticulitis without having a diverticulitis flare up, you will not experience any hardship.

A note on rectal bleeding. Anytime a person has this symptom, they should see a health care professional as soon as possible.

Treatment for Diverticulitis

Depending on your diagnosis, treatment at home may be all that's needed. Otherwise you may be hospitalized and even require surgery. If you are having symptoms, your doctor will check your abdomen for tenderness and then ask you about your bowel habits, diet, and any medicines you take. They may want to do some tests to screen for diverticular disease.

Diagnosing for actual diverticulosis is difficult because there are quite a few illnesses and conditions with similar symptoms such as irritable bowel syndrome (IBS). So your doctor may do some tests to be sure what condition you have.

Blood tests may be needed to rule out other medical conditions. A computed tomography (CT) scan will allow your doctor to see if you have pouches that are inflamed or infected. This is the most common diagnosing test for diverticulitis. An x-ray of organs in the abdomen may be included. A barium enema may also be done. The injected barium makes your colon more visible and easier to see. Your doctor may do a flexible sigmoidoscopy where a thin, flexible tube is inserted into your rectum. It's connected to a tiny video camera that will allow your doctor to look at your rectum and the last part of your colon.

And lastly, a colonoscopy may be required to see your entire large intestine. It is a procedure with a flexible tube with a tiny camera at the end called an endoscope. Because most people do not have symptoms, diverticulitis is often found through tests ordered for another problem like a colonoscopy to screen for cancer. A colonoscopy is often required to help evaluate pain or rectal bleeding.

In summary, your physician may order many of these tests to diagnose your problem.

Medication is sometimes prescribed if your physician diagnoses diverticulitis. For mild symptoms, you may be treated at home and your doctor is likely to recommend antibiotics, a liquid diet to start, and an over-the-counter pain reliever such as acetaminophen (Tylenol). Painkillers such as aspirin or ibuprofen should be avoided as they may upset the stomach and increase the risk of internal bleeding. As stated, antibiotics may be used to treat some cases. It's important to finish your antibiotics even if your symptoms get better.

Treatments for diverticulitis ALWAYS depends on the severity of the condition.

For example, with complicated diverticulitis, if you have a severe attack or have other health problems, you'll likely need to be hospitalized. Treatment can include intravenous antibiotics and/or insertion of a tube to drain an abscess which is a painful, swollen, infected and pus-filled area. About 25 percent of people with diverticulitis develop other complications such as a perforation, a small tear or hole in a pouch, peritonitis, an inflammation or infection of the lining of your abdomen, fistula, an abnormal passage between two organs and intestinal obstruction, a partial blockage of the movement of food or stool through your intestines.

If diverticulitis attacks are frequent or severe, the doctor may suggest surgery to remove a part of the patient's colon. If diverticula become infected, aggressive treatment may be needed. It can result in serious complications if left undetected. After treatment, your physician most likely will order a colonoscopy to make sure everything is in working order.

You may initially be diagnosed with diverticulosis or diverticulitis by your primary care provider (PCP). You may also see an emergency medicine specialist in a hospital's emergency department. In either case, you will likely be referred to a gastroenterologist, a specialist in the digestive tract, for treatment.

Summary

Treatment varies with your diagnosis. It ranges from at-home treatment to surgery depending on how severe the symptoms are. Tests may be ordered to find out how severe your diverticulitis is. Afterwards, a doctor will most likely order a colonoscopy to make sure everything's alright.

Causes of Diverticulitis

Doctors really aren't sure what causes diverticulitis. But commonly, they believe a low-fiber diet may play a part. For example, without much fiber, the colon has to work much harder to push a stool forward and the pressure causes weak spots. Bacteria grows in the pouches and this in turn can cause inflammation or infection. Although there is no clear evidence that not getting enough fiber in your diet is the cause of diverticulitis, the circumstantial evidence is quite convincing.

Diverticulitis is a "civilized disease". Today's Western diet most typically consists of highly processed foods, sugar and unhealthy fats. In places such as the United States, England and Australia diverticulitis is common. The disease first appeared in the United States in the early 1900's…approximately the same time when processed foods were first introduced. Diverticulitis is much less common in Asian and African countries where the typical diet is much higher in fiber.

In addition to a poor diet, other factors need to be considered such as age, obesity, smoking, a sedentary lifestyle, and a diet high in red meat and fat. Other possible causes for diverticulitis comprise of consuming dairy, lack of exercise, smoking and shortness of breath.

The bad news.

The disease affects from one-fourth to one-third of the population in developed countries. Several epidemiological studies have clearly shown that in the last decades the rates of clinic visits and hospital admissions for diverticulitis and its complications have progressively increased.

The good news.

Often diverticulitis flare ups can be reduced if not abolished. Maintaining a healthy balance of protein, fiber, with fresh fruits and vegetables is essential for keeping diverticulosis from flaring up.

No one knows exactly what causes diverticulitis but it's probably a combination of genetic and environmental influences. Risk factors include aging, weight gain, being male, and of course, having a diagnosis of diverticulosis.

Summary

I t's really not yet known what causes diverticulitis. But flare ups can be reduced if not abolished with a healthy, high fiber diet.

Foods to Avoid if You Suspect
Diverticulitis

Red Meat

Nowadays this is pretty obvious. Red meat is tougher and more difficult to digest unlike poultry or other white meat. It often further aggravates a stressed digestive tract.

Fatty Foods

This is good for all us trying to maintain a healthy diet but critical for those trying to avoid diverticulitis.

These type of foods will often provoke inflammation and slow down the healing of an infection. Unfortunately, this incudes cheese. Cheese is approximately 70 percent fat and for those suffering with chronic pain, cheese contains casein which is difficult to digest and often aggravates pain and bloating symptoms. Deep fried foods are a no-no. Chips, pizza, burgers, hotdogs, in other words, "junk food" will have to go!

Cruciferous Vegetables

Unlike most individuals on a high fiber diet, diverticulitis patients may find it valuable to not eat vegetables like cauliflower, broccoli, brussel sprouts, kale, cabbage, etc. Especially when eaten raw, such vegetables because of their high fiber content tend to produce gas. Alternatives might be cucumbers, celery, zucchini, squash and peppers. Talk to your doctor for a complete list on vegetables you might want to avoid.

Alcohol

Even for people without diverticulitis, alcohol puts much strain upon the gastrointestinal tract. For those with diverticulitis, it worsens the symptoms of diverticulitis, especially the pain and bloating. The flare ups can become more frequent. Alcohol can lead to dehydration and constipation. And if a person has a good diet but continues to consume alcohol, all their efforts are for naught. The flare ups will continue time and time again and will not give a chance for the body to heal.

Carbonated Beverages

Sodas and other bubbly drinks should be avoided. They can transform into an irritant often causing bloating. But diverticulitis patients are advised to consume as much fluid as possible, so check with your doctor to find other healthier options. Of course, drinking plain water is always best!

Nuts, Seeds, and Popcorn

For a long time, these were believed to be strictly prohibited. However, nowadays they are not. But they should be limited to prevent diverticulitis flare ups for often they can strain the gastrointestinal intestines, may worsen symptoms, and slow down healing. Immediately after a flare up these should be **avoided** because of their high fiber content including peanut butter. Work with you doctor. These can easily be reintroduced once you're recovered.

As always even after the flare up has passed, if nuts cause any discomfort you should avoid them. No matter how healthy their reputation may be. The seeds in tomatoes, zucchini, cucumbers, strawberries, raspberries along with poppy seeds are usually easy tolerate. But monitor your body's response to any food as we are all individuals and these may not be good for your systems as well.

Whole Grains

If you have acute diverticulitis, your doctor may suggest avoiding these. They are usually a healthy choice for diverticulitis sufferers because of their fiber and being good for overall colon wellbeing. So check with your doctor before consuming these!

Spicy Foods

Spicy foods can cause distress to the rectal area and obstruct easy bowel movements. They can trigger episodes of diverticulitis and patients are often asked to avoid cuisines such as Indian and Thai.

Dairy Products

Whether or not we are lactose intolerant, dairy products often cause digestion issues. Bloating is a common side effect. Patients with diverticulitis should often choose lactose-free yogurt and soy or almond milk. With diverticulitis, it's often more difficult to digest lactose (a sugar found in cow's milk).

Cheese should be avoided at all costs not only because it's a dairy product but also high in fat. Unfortunately too, those with diverticulitis should steer clear of butter. Try oil spreads or olive spreads that cause no reaction.

Corn

Corn is often the underlying cause of digestive problems because corn is high in sugar as well. It plays a part in symptomatic diverticular disease. You should give this vegetable up entirely, cut back or opt for the processed cream corn which has lower amounts of fiber and sugars as well. But be on the lookout for symptoms regardless of which manner you choose!

Summary

For diverticulitis patients the choice is yours. Some types of food may be harder to give up than others. You can experiment with some types of food to see what your limit is. And any refined sugar is bad too like white sugar, brown sugar, cane sugar and corn syrup. If you only get sugar from fruit it's ideal. However, if you do choose a sweetener go for honey, maple syrup or dates.

One good thing. Diverticulitis is a condition that forces you to watch your diet! A benefit for anyone.

Foods to Eat During and After a
Diverticulitis Flare Up

If you have been diagnosed with diverticulitis, your physician will put you on a clear liquid diet. It's very restrictive and gives your body a chance to heal. It's imperative that you follow the right diet. The goal is to decrease fecal bulk and this in turn will ease the inflammation. So even though this diet is no fun it will help you heal faster!

A liquid diet could have recommendations such as: chicken, vegetable, or bone broth; ice chips; water; plain gelatin; tea; light colored hard candies; light colored juice; strained lemonade. Soothing ginger tea is a good beverage to sip on. Ginger has been used for thousands of years for medicinal purposes to reduce nausea and pain.

Juicing fruits and vegetables can definitely give you a boost. Carrots, beets, grapes, apples, lettuce and watercress can all be enjoyed. Fruits should be peeled and not have the skin of course. Until your health care provider recommends it, you should avoid foods high in fiber! Again, this includes foods with tough skins and small seeds.

As you get better, you will soon be able to consume more solid foods. Again, your physician will probably give you a list of what you can have and what to avoid. You can add fiber-rich foods but do it slowly and listen to your body. Prepare all foods so that they're tender. Try to avoid roasting, broiling and grilling. Fruits and vegetables (if they are not cruciferous) can be added and unrefined grains such as quinoa, black rice, and fermented grains.

This can't be said enough! Listen to your body! If you develop symptoms, your doctor may return to the full-liquid diet. It may take a few months but be patient. Your health is at stake.

When you're ready to add foods high in fiber, that it's never good to add such foods all at once! Add one new food every three or four days. Then you can begin to consume about 25-35 grams of fiber each day to not have any more potential diverticulitis flare ups. Add in some potatoes, sweet potatoes, and oats. Your physician may list the things most likely you can eat and foods you should avoid based on your condition.

Foods high in fiber with a concentration on soluble fibers and a little lighter on insoluble fibers is good for diverticulitis patients. Soluble fiber is a plant fiber that does not dissolve, it actually forms as a gel when mixed with liquids. Foods high in soluble fiber include oatmeal, nuts, beans, apples, and blueberries.
Insoluble fiber is known for its roughage or bulk qualities. Foods to look for that are high in insoluble fiber are the seeds and skins of fruit and vegetables as well as whole-wheat bread and brown rice. But if foods

high in insoluble fiber are uncomfortable for diverticulitis patients, one can always boost soluble fiber. Some tips to get more fiber…use beans to top your salad, always snack on fruits and vegetables and always make your grains whole grains. No more white bread! If you're having trouble getting enough fiber from foods it may be OK with your doctor for you to take a fiber supplement like psyllium fiber.

While it's not possible to cure diverticulitis, you can prevent flare ups by eating healthy, high fiber foods. And always be sure to drink plenty of fluids! Remember, good old water is best!

Summary

Depending on your symptoms your physician may put you on a clear liquid diet to let your body heal. As your body recovers, you will move to a diet where you can consume soft food, a low fiber diet. And finally, you will be ready for a high fiber diet.

Lifestyle Changes

Diverticulitis requires more than just changing your diet to aid in a healthy digestive tract. Switch to a healthy high fiber diet. While you are enjoying your food, remember that digestion begins in the mouth. **Eat slowly. It is essential to chew each bite of food until it is nearly liquefied.** The more you break down the food...the more nutrients are ready to be absorbed.

Other suggestions include:

- Exercise daily. Running or brisk walking will help reduce flare ups and relieve symptoms. Exercise also reduces stress and supports a healthy weight. Try to exercise 30 minutes daily.
- As in life, even without diverticulosis, your psychological health is essential. Learn how to manage and cope with daily stress.
- Avoid straining on the toilet. To reduce this elevate the feet slightly using a stool.
- Drink plenty of fluids. Fiber can be constipating. But if you drink enough, you will replace what's absorbed by the fiber and consequently increase the soft, bulky waste in your colon.

- Practice mindfulness and meditation. When we are focused and are more peaceful, it can boost the immune system and help in healing the body.
- Start your day with lemon water and end it with light, not potent, ginger tea.

Some Supplements to Treat Diverticulitis

Always ask your physician if you can use any of the following.

- Slippery Elm. Native Americans have used this to aid in digestive problems. It is often recommended to relieve symptoms of GERD, Crohn's Disease, IBS, and more.
- Aloe. In a juice form this can help in digestion and standardizes bowels.
- Licorice Root. This helps lower stomach acid levels, can relieve heartburn, and act as a mild laxative.

Suggested Questions to
Ask Your Doctor

When you see your doctor after having been diagnosed with diverticulitis, the following questions are suggestions for you to ask. But always incorporate your own! It's very beneficial to have a written list so you can record the answers as well as not forget to ask your questions.

- How serious is this condition?
- What causes diverticular disease?
- What is the treatment for diverticular disease?
- Will tests be required?
- Will surgery be necessary?
- Are there foods that should be avoided?
- Are there foods that are recommended?
- How can I tell if I am getting enough fiber in my diet?
- How will I know if I am getting too much fiber in my diet?
- Would seeing a dietician for an eating plan help?
- How effective is diet in controlling this disease?
- Is there a cure for diverticulitis?
- What are some simple steps for increasing the fiber intake of my meals?
- Should I eat one type of fiber more than another?

Steps to Help Manage Diverticulitis

No foods are known to trigger diverticulitis attacks. And no special diet is known to prevent attacks.

Usually the pain goes away pretty quickly with diverticulitis. Your doctor may want to see you that same week to make sure you're improving. And a colonoscopy may be done about six weeks later after your symptoms are under control to check for any other problems like colon cancer. Remember too, to completely heal, it may sometimes take three months to a year before you can go on a diet with high fiber foods. Be patient! You will feel better the rest of your life.

Most diverticulitis treatments work but those diverticula remain always in your intestines. You could get diverticulitis again. To prevent a diverticulitis flare up and to avoid constipation it's important to:

- Get enough fiber.
- Keep hydrated.
- Go to the bathroom when you feel the urge to go.
- Exercise regularly.

Diverticulitis Consists of
Three Diet Phases

In treating diverticulitis depending on your symptoms of course, your physician will put you on a Clear Liquid Diet (Phase One), a Low Fiber Diet (Phase Two) and finally, a High Fiber Diet (Phase Three). If everything goes smoothly, you will soon be able to eat a High Fiber Diet. However, if you experience any symptoms, your physician may return you to a previous diet phase. For example, if you have problems with the Low Fiber Diet (Phase One), you could go back on a Clear Liquid Diet (Phase One) until you can tolerate low fiber foods.

Each Phase follows with a listing of foods for that specific phase. This guidebook ends with suggested recipes for each diet phase.

Summary

Phase One helps you recover from a diverticulitis flare up, Phase Two helps your body move towards a normal diet, and Phase Three is the third and least restrictive diet that you can eat once your body is up to it, offering you as much freedom as possible without the risk of a flare up occurring.

Phase One:

Foods for a Clear Liquid Diet

Follow your physician's instruction to the letter! It will help you to get well quicker. Most liquid diets consist of:

- Broth
- Clear soda
- Fruit juices without pulp
- Ice chips
- Ice pops without bits of fruit or fruit pulp
- Plain gelatin
- Plain water
- Tea or coffee without cream

Clear liquids mean just that. You must be able to see through them. This diet is short-term for digestive problems and surgery. Clear liquids help keep you hydrated, provides some needed electrolytes and gives you some energy when you cannot eat solid food. Liquid diets can become monotonous. To lessen the monotony, alternate between cold and hot. Use different type of fruit juices and ice pops to and try to vary the colors of your meals and snacks. These simple tips can help in continuing one's appetite. This diet is not exciting but remember you will not be on it forever! A typical menu on a clear liquid diet follows.

Breakfast:
- 1 glass pulp-free fruit juice
- 1 bowl gelatin
- 1 cup of coffee or tea, without dairy products

Lunch
- 1 glass pulp-free fruit juice
- 1 glass water
- 1 cup broth
- 1 bowl gelatin

Dinner
- 1 cup pulp-free juice or water
- 1 cup broth (chicken, beef, or bone)
- 1 bowl gelatin
- 1 cup coffee or tea, without dairy products

Snacks
- 1 glass fruit juice (pulp-free)
- 1 bowl gelatin
- 1 pulp-free ice pop
- 1 cup coffee or tea, without dairy products, or a soft drink

Phase Two:

A Low Residue/Low Fiber Diet

People who have <u>diverticulitis</u> are usually advised to eat a low fiber diet and sometimes a low residue diet. A low fiber diet includes refined breads, crackers, cereals, pasta, white rice, and low fiber vegetables and fruits (with no skin, seeds or pulp), very limited milk products (if at all!), well-cooked lean proteins, and eggs.

Both limit the amount of dietary fiber and residue-producing food in the diet. Dietary fiber, which is found in plant foods, cannot be digested; residue is the undigested part of plants that contribute to stool. Limiting dietary fiber and residue reduces the amount of food that passes through the large intestine.

Although a low residue diet and low fiber diet are used interchangeably, a low residue diet is more RESTRICTIVE than a low fiber diet. While the low fiber diet allows some fresh fruits (without peels or seeds of course), the low residue diet does NOT allow any raw fruits. Check with your physician on which one is necessary.

Phase Two:

Foods for a Transitional Low Fiber Diet

After a clear liquid diet, the following food groups gives you an idea of what your physician might suggest you eat.

Food Groups

Meats:
Chicken, turkey, fish, tender cuts of beef and pork, ground meats, skinless hot dogs, sausage patties without whole spices, eggs.

Fruits and Juices:
Fruit juices without pulp, banana, avocado, applesauce, canned peaches and pears, cooked fruit without the skin/seeds.

Vegetables:
Well-cooked or canned vegetables, potatoes without skin, tomato sauces, vegetable juice. Best to avoid cruciferous vegetables.

Cereals and Grains:
Low-fiber dry or cooked cereals (with almond/soy milk), white rice, pasta, macaroni, or noodles.

Breads and Crackers:
White/refined breads and rolls, toast, plain crackers, graham crackers.

Desserts:
Plain cake, sherbet, gelatin, fruit whips.

Herbs and Spices:
All ground spices or herbs. (No whole spices such as peppercorns, whole cloves, celery seeds!)

Dairy:
Best to not have it. Use lactose free or low lactose for milk, cheese, yogurt, butter, etc. Olive oil for cooking. Live like you are lactose intolerant.

Phase Two: Recommended Equipment for a Low Fiber Diet

Most foods can be adapted to meet your needs with a Low Fiber Diet. Many main dishes, such as noodles, stews, and casseroles can be put into a blender with some liquid. Add liquid until the food is the right consistency. Here is some equipment that you may find helpful:

Blender: Can be used for all types of food and are excellent for soups and shakes. It requires liquid for the right consistency.

Food processor: This is the most expensive item of all the equipment, but it is good for shredding, slicing, chopping or blending foods.

Hand-held blender: This is a convenient because you can use it purée your favorite soups right in the pot. It can also be used to soften well-cooked foods in a small bowl for 1 or 2 portions.

Household mesh strainer or sieve: Tool for straining fruits and vegetables but not meats.

Food mill: This is an excellent tool to strain fruits, vegetables, and soups, but do not use it with meats.

Phase Three: Foods for a High Fiber Diet

Today, it is thought that a high fiber diet and clean food are best for us. Therefore, you're very lucky when you switch to a high fiber diet. There are multiple cookbooks and recipes to be found! And always have the ingredients in the house to toss together a healthy, colorful salad. No longer is a salad just a wedge of lettuce with a piece of tomato. If you have high fiber food in your home, you won't be tempted to order out for junk food either! Have fun discovering how to make your favorite recipes new again and healthy!

Most fruits such as pears, apples, bananas, oranges, figs, raisins, etc. are high in fiber. *If tolerated*, those with seeds such as raspberries and strawberries, are OK. Most vegetables are OK too except for the cruciferous vegetables such as cauliflower, broccoli, brussel sprouts, kale, cabbage, etc. And remember…AVOID CORN!

Try to eat whole grains, cereal and pasta. This will include whole-wheat bread and pasta, barley, bran, oatmeal, brown rice, etc. If anything doesn't agree with your digestive system, give it up and find a replacement. Review the foods to avoid list. Patients with diverticulitis, and even most people, cannot eat everything! Find something else you enjoy as a replacement. This food may eventually become a favorite.

Recipes for the
Three Diverticulitis Diet Phases

Note: All of the following use U.S. measuring standards. Convert to metric.

Phase One: Clear Liquid Recipes

Bone Broth

Bone broth is very trendy and yes, you can buy it. But it is very expensive and somewhat easy to make your own! The recipe that follows was inspired by Bon Appétit Magazine.

A real bone broth is made with bones and cuts of meat high in collagen, like marrow, knuckles, and feet. Get to know your butcher! (And now I understand why my Aunt always saved the bones after a chicken or roast!) While beef is the meat most people associate with bone broth, it can also be made with lamb, pork, chicken, veal, and more. Blanch your bones first. Cover the bones with cold water, bring to a boil, and let them cook at an aggressive simmer for 20 minutes before draining and roasting. This will help take off the unsightly grizzle or meat left on the bones.

Then roast your bones. Roasting browns and caramelizes the bones. Set the oven temperature up high to 450°. Check constantly until the bones are "done". The next step is to actually boil the bones. Do not waste the crisped brown bits on the bottom of the pan; loosen them with a little water and a metal spatula, and add those to your stockpot. Doing this adds a lot of flavor!

Ingredients:
A good bone broth doesn't need much more than the bones, onion, and garlic. This is not the time to get rid of all your "stuff" in the refrigerator!

Instructions:
Femur bones are big. Use the biggest, heaviest stockpot you've got, and fill it up with your roasted bones, plus the other ingredients based on your taste. Add just enough water to cover the bones, bring to a boil, lower the heat to a simmer, and cover. The bone-to-water ratio should be close enough that the resulting broth is intensely flavored. The bones should not be floating. This will make the bone broth taste "watered down".

Cover the pot and bring to a gentle boil. Reduce heat to a very low simmer and cook with lid slightly ajar, skimming foam and excess fat occasionally, for at least 8 hours. The more it simmers the better. Add more water if necessary.

After it simmers for quite a while, remove the pot from the heat and let cool slightly. Strain the broth using a fine-mesh sieve. Discard bones and vegetables. Let continue to cool until barely warm.

Do not ever put hot broth in the refrigerator! Put into smaller containers. It will stay good for about three days, and freeze up to three months. To have smaller portions for later, put the broth in ice cube trays.

And pat yourself on the back! For you made your own bone broth!

Chicken Broth

Ingredients:
- 1/3 cup chicken broth concentrate
- 8 cups water
- 4 stalks chopped celery
- 1 whole chopped onion
- 2 large chopped carrots
- 4 cloves smashed garlic
- 4 Tbsp. unflavored gelatin

Instructions:
Add chicken concentrate to water. Add remaining ingredients. Bring to a boil then add gelatin.

Reduce heat and simmer for 30-45 minutes. Strain vegetables and reserve broth. It tastes better when you make your own broth!

Coconut Lime Cooler

Ingredients:
- 2 cup coconut water
- 2 tsp. organic lime juice

Instructions:
Add chilled coconut water and lime juice to a glass with ice. Garnish with a lime wedge. Easy when you don't want to go to the trouble of juicing or blending!

Phase Two: Low Fiber Recipes

Non-Dairy Cream of Wheat

Ingredients:
- 3 Tbsp. instant dry cream of wheat
- 1 ¼ cups canned coconut milk

Instructions:
Make the cream of wheat according to package directions substituting coconut milk for the water. Drizzle with honey.

Green Smoothie

The green smoothie seems to be all the rage. And it's a wonderful way to get your vegetables! Try the following but experiment to your own taste. Yum!

Ingredients:
- 1 Tbsp. fresh ginger (~1 small knob, skin removed)
- 1/2 lemon or lime, juiced (1 Tbsp.)
- 1/3 cup light coconut milk
- 1 1/2 cups chopped frozen pineapple (as ripe as possible!)
- 1 small ripe frozen banana, previously peeled, sliced and frozen
- 1 large handful spinach
- 1 small handful kale
- 2/3 cup unsweetened plain almond milk
- 3/4 cup water

Instructions:

Add all ingredients to blender and blend thoroughly on high speed until completely smooth. If it isn't quite blending, add a bit more water or almond milk. Blend well especially the ginger. Serve over ice. Store leftovers in refrigerator for up to 24 hours. However, this is always best when fresh!

Blueberry Smoothie

Ingredients:
- 1 cup cranberry juice
- 1 cup silken tofu, soy or other non-dairy milk
- 2 cups frozen blueberries
- 2 tablespoons honey or maple syrup

Instructions:
Mix all ingredients in a blender a minute at high speed until smooth and frothy.

Easy Unsweetened Applesauce

Ingredients:
- 4 lbs. skinned apples
- 1/2 cup of water
- 2 tsp cinnamon
- nutmeg, vanilla or mixed spice (optional)

Instructions:
Skin, core and slice your apples. Add cinnamon and other spices, if desired. Cook the apples with a splash of water on medium heat for 20 minutes until soft and mushy. Puree with a hand-held blender or in your food processor. This applesauce will keep in the fridge for 1 week. Much better than store-bought!

Low Fiber Vegetable Chicken Soup

Ingredients:

- 5 cups chicken broth
- 1 carrot
- 1 potato
- 1/2 cup tomato flesh (no skin or seeds)
- 1 bunch asparagus tips
- 1/2 cup cooked small pasta

Instructions:

Place broth, carrot and potato in a small saucepan. Bring to a boil, then reduce heat and cook until vegetables are very tender. Add tomatoes and asparagus tips and cook until asparagus is tender. Stir in cooked pasta and cook until heated through.

Low Fiber Carrot and Beet Soup

Ingredients:
- 4 cups vegetable broth
- 1 carrot, sliced
- 1 can cooked beets (not pickled)

Instructions:
Put sliced carrot and vegetable broth in a small saucepan. Bring to a boil, reduce heat, cook, covered, until carrots are very tender. Add beets. Cook until heated through. Puree until smooth.

Butternut Squash Soup

Ingredients
- 1 - 10 ounce package frozen squash, thawed
- 2/3 cup unsweetened light coconut milk
- 3/4 cup water
- 1/2 teaspoon cinnamon
- 1 teaspoon dried parsley
- 1 tablespoon green onions, chopped

Instructions:
Place all of the ingredients into a blender or food processor and puree until smooth. Place soup in a saucepan and warm over medium heat. Enjoy!

Easy Low Fiber Chicken Risotto

Ingredients:
- 2 tablespoons olive oil
- 2 garlic cloves, crushed
- 1 medium brown onion, diced
- 1 medium carrot, diced
- 2 cups white rice
- 5 cups vegetable liquid stock
- 1 medium zucchini, chopped
- 1 small roasted chicken, meat removed and chopped

Instructions:
Heat oil in heavy-based pan over medium heat. Add garlic, onion and carrot and cook, stirring, until vegetables are softened. Add rice and cook, stirring, for 1 minute or until lightly coated in oil. Add 2 cups of the stock and bring to boil. Cover and simmer for 6-8 minutes or until liquid is absorbed. Continue to add remaining stock approximately one-half cup at a time, along with the zucchini and chicken. Cook, stirring constantly, for 8-10 minutes or until liquid is absorbed and rice is tender.

Baked Halibut

Ingredients:
- 2 lbs. halibut fillets
- 1 cup Italian breadcrumbs
- 2 tsp. chopped parsley
- 1/4 cup melted butter (if not tolerated, margarine)
- 1/2 tsp. garlic powder

Instructions:
Clean and pat dry fillets with a paper towel. In medium bowl, mix together breadcrumbs, melted butter or margarine, garlic powder, chopped parsley. Coat the fillets. Shallow-fry the fillets in a heated pan for two to five minutes on each side. When done serve with parsley.

Spinach Stir-Fry with Garlic

Ingredients:
- 16 oz. baby spinach
- 2 cloves garlic, finely chopped
- ¼ cup chicken broth

Instructions:
Preheat a medium safe nonstick pan over medium heat. Add broth and chopped garlic.

Stir with a wooden spoon until fragrant (two to three minutes). Add spinach and sauté three to five minutes. Hate raw spinach? Cook it!

Slow Cooker Mashed Sweet Potatoes

Ingredients:
- 4 medium sweet potatoes
- 1/4 tsp. nutmeg
- 3 tsp. ground cinnamon
- 1 Tbsp. coconut oil

Instructions:
Wash potatoes and prick with a fork. Combine coconut oil, cinnamon and nutmeg. Coat each potato with mixture. Place in slow cooker with ½ cup water. Cook on low four to six hours, or until tender when pierced. Remove skin and mash.

No-Chocolate 'Brownies'

Ingredients:
- 1 1/2 cups grated carrots
- 2 eggs
- 1 cup vegetable oil
- 1/2 cup unsweetened applesauce
- 1 3/4 cup regular oatmeal
- 1 tsp. baking soda
- 1 tsp. cinnamon
- 1 cup loosely packed raisins

Preheat oven to 350°

In one bowl mix dry ingredients.
- 1 1/4 cup regular oatmeal ground into flour (use a food processor)
- 1/2 cup regular oatmeal
- 1 tsp cinnamon
- 1 tsp baking soda
- 1 cup raisins

In another bowl mix wet ingredients.
- 1 1/2 cups grated carrots
- 2 large eggs
- ½ cup vegetable oil
- ½ cup unsweetened applesauce

Add dry ingredients to the wet and mix until blended completely. Let sit for about 5 minutes until liquid is absorbed. Drop by measured tablespoons onto parchment lined cookie sheets. Bake for approximately 15 - 18 minutes until firm and golden brown in color. Remove from pan and cool on a wire rack. Yum!

Recommended Equipment
for a Low Fiber Diet

Most foods can be adapted to meet your needs with a Low Fiber Diet. Many main dishes, such as noodles, stews, and casseroles can be put into a blender with some liquid. Add liquid until the food is the right consistency. Here is some equipment that you may find helpful:

Blender: Can be used for all types of food and are excellent for soups and shakes. It requires liquid for the right consistency.

Food processor: This is the most expensive item of all the equipment, but it is good for shredding, slicing, chopping or blending foods.

Hand-held blender: This is a convenient because you can use it purée your favorite soups right in the pot. It can also be used to soften well-cooked foods in a small bowl for 1 or 2 portions.

Household mesh strainer or sieve: Tool for straining fruits and vegetables but not meats.

Food mill: This is an excellent tool to strain fruits, vegetables, and soups, but do not use it with meats.

Phase Three: High Fiber Diet Recipes

Overnight Oatmeal

Ingredients:
- ⅓ cup old-fashioned rolled oats
- ⅓ cup unsweetened coconut milk beverage
- ⅓ cup dried apricots
- 1 Tbsp. hazelnuts
- 1 tsp. maple syrup

Instructions:
Mix together oats and coconut milk in a jar or bowl. Cover and refrigerate overnight. In the morning, heat if desired. Top with apricots, hazelnuts and maple syrup.

Healthy High-Fiber Hummus Sandwich

Ingredients:
- 2 slices whole-grain bread
- 5 tablespoons hummus (any flavor!)
- ½ cup mixed salad greens
- ¼ medium red bell pepper cut into strips
- ¼ cup sliced cucumber
- ¼ cup shredded carrot

Instructions:
Spread hummus on bread. Fill with ingredients. Sandwich can be refrigerated up to 4 hours.

Chicken Pasta with Veggies

Ingredients:

- 8 oz. spaghetti
- 2 cloves crushed garlic
- 2 Tbsp. olive oil
- Sliced medium onion
- 2 skinless chicken breast cut into bite-size pieces
- 2 cups broccoli
- 2 cups cauliflower
- 2 cups julienne carrots
- 2 Tbsp. soy sauce

Instructions:

Cook pasta in boiling water per directions. Meanwhile, heat oil in a large skillet or wok over medium-high heat. Cook garlic in oil for 1 minute. Stir in onion, and cook until soft. Stir in chicken, and cook until done. Mix in the broccoli, cauliflower, and carrots, and cook for 2 to 5 minutes, stirring frequently. Season with soy sauce.Toss pasta with vegetables and serve warm.

Pork with Pears

Ingredients:

- 2 pork tenderloins
- 2 thinly sliced garlic cloves
- 1 Tbsp. minced fresh thyme
- 1 Tbsp. olive oil
- 4 cored and quartered Bartlett pears

Instructions:

Preheat oven to 475 degrees. Cut 10 small slits in each tenderloin and fill with garlic and thyme. In ovenproof skillet heat oil. Add pork until browned on both sides. Add pears to skillet. Cook until pork registers 145 degrees, about 10 minutes. Let rest 5 minutes. Slice pork and serve with pears and pan juices.

Deluxe Trail Mix

Ingredients:
- 1 cup puffed quinoa or puffed millet
- 1/4 cups unsweetened coconut flakes
- 1/2 cup whole roasted almonds
- 1/2 cup raw cashews
- 1/2 cup dried banana chips (broken in half)
- 1/4 cup chopped dried mango, papaya or cherries
- 2 tablespoons candied ginger

Instructions:
In a medium mixing bowl, toss all ingredients together until evenly combined. Store in an airtight container for up to 1 month. This is easy and good to have on hand, Feel free to use any kind of nuts if they agree with you. Experiment and use what you like!

Lemon Coconut No-Bake Nibbles

Ingredients:
- 8 pitted dates
- 1/2 cup unsweetened applesauce
- Zest and juice of 1 large lemon
- 1/2 tsp vanilla extract
- 1/2 cup coconut flour
- 1/4 cup almond milk (more if needed)
- 1/2 cup unsweetened shredded coconut

Instructions:
Place dates, applesauce, lemon juice, lemon zest, and vanilla in a large food processor. Process until dates look nearly pureed and mixture is combined. Add coconut flour. Process until mixture forms a smooth ball of "dough". Roll into 12 balls. Place coconut in a small bowl and roll balls. Store in an air-tight container in the refrigerator.

Last Words on Diverticulitis

I hope this handbook convinced you what a serious disease diverticulitis can be. So change your eating habits! Remember the diverticulitis diet phases. Try the recipes or modify your own. Feel free to experiment. In the end, try to eat a high fiber diet. And remember, after all, eating is a joy of life. Relish and savor your food. Bon appétit!

Printed in Great Britain
by Amazon

46886223R00036